Praise for *Pause, Rest, Be*

"In need of an inner reset? Look no further than *Pause, Rest, Be*. Octavia's wise and honest teachings put the reader at ease and give us permission to embrace more of our true self than we ever thought possible."

—Light Watkins, author of *Knowing Where to Look*

"It's not an exaggeration to say that *Pause, Rest, Be* is life changing. Like a restorative backward bend, our heart opens and heals with the support of Octavia Raheem's words. This book is like a song and could be called 'Octavia's Gita.' How lucky we are to hear her siren song, drawing us back to the truth of our essential self."

—Jivana Heyman, author of *Accessible Yoga* and *Yoga Revolution*

"A sacred call inward—home to yourself. *Pause, Rest, Be* is a poetic prayer of real-life wisdom, and the depth of stillness is felt on the page. Octavia's words are a soothing invitation for us to courageously do what most of us fiercely resist: slowing down, letting go, and listening. Whether you are mourning the loss of an old life, in the midst of vast uncertainty, or beginning a new chapter, this book will support you to soften, feel, rest, and move closer to the truth of who you are."

—Shannon Algeo, author of *Trust Your Truth*

"For those of us who carry the weight of the world on our shoulders and in our hearts, Octavia Raheem's words offer a call to rest that is not about denial or selfishness but is instead about the rest that is required if we are to live fully and embrace the complexity of our shared humanity. *Pause, Rest, Be* is an antidote to a culture of speed and burnout (often rooted in trauma) and a call to remember who we really are and can be."

—Hala Khouri, MA, SEP, E-RYT, author of *Peace from Anxiety*

Pause, Rest, Be

*Stillness Practices
for Courage
in Times of Change*

Octavia F. Raheem

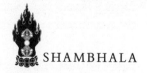

SHAMBHALA

Shambhala Publications, Inc.
2129 13th Street
Boulder, Colorado 80302
www.shambhala.com

Cover design: Shubhani Sarkar
Author photo: LC Morrissette
Interior design: Greta D. Sibley

9 8 7 6 5 4 3 2

Printed in the United States of America

Shambhala Publications makes every effort to print on acid-free, recycled
paper.
Shambhala Publications is distributed worldwide by Penguin
Random House, Inc., and its subsidiaries.

Library of Congress Cataloging-in-Publication Data
Names: Raheem, Octavia F., author.
Title: Pause, rest, be: stillness practices for courage in times of change /
Octavia F. Raheem.
Description: Boulder, Colorado: Shambhala Publications, Inc., [2022]
Identifiers: LCCN 2021018007 | ISBN 9781611809855 (trade paperback)
Subjects: LCSH: Self-actualization (Psychology) | Motivation (Psychology) |
Mind and body—Religious aspects.
Classification: LCC BF637.S4 R236 2022 | DDC 158.1—dc23
LC record available at https://lccn.loc.gov/2021018007

For everyone who survived the last few years.

And everyone who didn't.

Contents

Acknowledgments

To My Beloveds,

Jemar Raheem, my husband, your dedication to our love story provides me space to write, revise, and edit as I please. For making sure wherever we are together is home. For being shelter from storms. For walking alongside and sometimes carrying me through endings, in between spaces, and beginnings.

Oyetunde Raheem, my son, thank you for your innate way of knowing when "Mama is listening for something deep and that's why she's gone away and being real quiet."

To My Mothers,

Millie Miller, your love is soil. Your light, nourishment. Your prayers, holy water. My discipline and devotion, my faith and courage, is a harvest from the seeds you tirelessly tended within me. This book is only one piece of fruit, a single and beautiful flower in your garden. For growing with me.

Angela Strickland, my mother-in-love, your story and mine begin in the same place. For the grace, love, softness, and strength to write and rewrite as many beginnings as we can imagine. For understanding beyond words. For sharing your story with me.

Gail Parker, for making tracks on this road that I could follow in, for holding the sacred rest space for me to break open and be put back together—again and again, for leading with your brave heart, for telling our truth.

To My Sisters,

Ebony A. Reynolds, I will never forget how you took your summer job money one year and paid my way to writing camp. You believed in me before I believed in myself. For seeing me.

Women of Devoted to Rest 2021, you lived this book before it was born. Your breath is woven into every page here. For investing in my work. For resting with me.

Michelle C. Johnson, your generous heart gave me courage to begin this project.

Tiffany Johnson and Rashida Parrish, my book models, for showing us all what claiming rest as a birthright can look like in our bodies. For allowing your whole selves to be seen.

To LeeAnn C. Morrissette, my photographer, for lending me and all who lay their eyes on this book, your eyes.

To My Seers,

Shana Nunnelly, you read and remembered the future. It is here. More is coming. For sharing your gifts of Spirit.

Tracy Jennings-Hill, you said this was already written in the stars. For sharing the secrets of the old sky.

Iya Ayorinde & Nini, for every chant song, prayer divined, and offering made on my behalf.

To My Teachers,
Dr. Gail Parker, Maya Breuer, Tracee Stanley, Chanti Tacoronte-Perez, Gina Minyard, Graham Fowler, and Swami Premajyoti Saraswati for teaching me how to nourish my destiny. For graciously sharing tools that help me understand my purpose and unlock the courage to live more freely within it.

To My Editors and Support Team,
Beth Frankl, for answering the call. For every response. For rooting for me and this book before I'd written a single word. For filling in the cracks with your gold.

Emily Coughlin, for sharing your skillful precision and doing so with ease.

Diedre Hammons, for your keen eye and early affirmation of the goodness within this book.

Brook Blander, for your magic and the reminders to both share freely and protect the red clayness in my voice, always.

Jivana Heyman, you heard what I was afraid to say, for listening and responding anyway.

Acknowledgments

To My Ancestors,

Thank you for trusting me with your dreams.

To my late father, Charles E. Ramsey III, for reaching from beyond and holding my hand as I wrote.

I bow. I offer immense gratitude to you all.

To you, holding this book right now, thank you.

Introduction

In many ways, I've been front-lining my life the last few years.
I've been in the trenches of my own being.

I've charged ahead over many landscapes and vast fields.

The field of endings and the confusion and clinging that often
accompanies them. The landscape of new beginnings and the
uncertainty and excitement that come along with them. I've
rushed through and forced something—anything—to be next.
I also lingered at that place in between, that liminal space, that
point that is not an end or a beginning. It's the edge of both.

So much of it felt like a battle. I've yielded a formidable sword
against it all.

I've been a devoted warrior, hoping that every fight strengthens
me for my future. I've been a dedicated student, trying to

trust that no matter how challenging or painful a lesson is, it transforms into healing wisdom for me. I have faced inner and outer enemies who were Goliath. In the face of giants, my five-foot-one self didn't back down or look for an escape.

For so long, I've relied solely on the trinity of hard work, grit, and relentlessness.

This holy trinity has served me well and, at the same time, left me weary and tired. My little slingshot is broken. The handle of my sword is worn. I put down my armor. In this place of bone-deep exhaustion, I surrender and lay down. There is a time and place to push, hustle, and grind. I've always lived my life in that way and from that place. Perhaps you have too. Yet, here I am in a new place. To access the wisdom needed now, I must be still. A movement is coming, and, first, we must be still.

Now is no ordinary moment in time. Now is a place of startling individual and collective endings. Now is the space before something else becomes. Now is both a promise and fulfillment of fresh beginnings. The sacred cycle of being human seems to be speeding up. For many, we assume the remedy is to match that speed. As we become more and more exhausted, anxious, and disillusioned with trying to keep up with an inhumane pace, it is apparent that all of the battling, the swiftness, and the forging ahead brought me—brought us—collectively to this moment.

This moment where we are perhaps finally ready to listen for a new rhythm and tune.

Listen. We are descending into quiet. Being thrown into it, really. I hear a sound so striking in its silence that it has displaced us all. It has put us in our place.

Human.
Be. Still.

We can no longer outrun this without collectively slowing down. We cannot profit from this without the bottom meticulously falling out. We cannot package, sell, or otherwise capitalize on this without paying with our very own lives.

We can no longer live in the way that so many of us have learned to be:

Individual
Grinding
Hustling
Calculating
Competitive
Consumed with work
Away from our families while saying . . . family matters.

We cannot outrun this. The only way to beat this is to stop. Now. And still, some of us may lose.

There can be no screaming match here. If we keep yelling over everything and everybody, we will miss it.

So, stop. Really, really stop. Go read. write. rest. take care. paint. cry. dance. love. sit in the rain. grieve. reconnect to the source of your strength. cook at home. call your elders. pray. love. be transformed.

Please stop spinning. Please stop scrambling to be productive in the way that mattered yesterday.

Honor the lessons of yesterday and let everything else about that recent, yet distant past fall away.

Something is happening now that demands we be present for it.

If we keep going like nothing is happening, we will miss it.

It—the world that is ending and the one that is coming.

It—this space in between.

I've seen glimpses of *it* in my dreams.

Beloveds, *it* gets worse. My God, *it* does.

We get better. My God, we get better.

And then . . . hallelujah. Glory.

It.

It gets better as we get better.

It gets so much better.

Arundhati Roy reminds us, "Another world is possible."

We are descending into quiet.

Listen.

––––––––

I created *Pause, Rest, Be* to meet you in the places that shape, redefine, and sometimes undo us: endings, liminal space, and beginnings. The places of falling aparts and mergings. Of letting go and coming together. Union. This book contains my personal reflections on endings, the place in between, and beginnings. It is also a book of inquiry and practice. Each section ends with a prayer that crosses faiths to reach all hearts.

It is a place to practice less asana and cultivate a relationship with embodied rest as a tool of reflection.

We will explore the following restorative or resting poses that will allow us to feel held, cradled, and protected (*so necessary right now*) before reading each short chapter:

> The end—Corpse Pose
> The space in between—Side-Lying Pose
> The place of beginnings—Child's Pose

––––––––

Restorative yoga is a practice that invites us to be at home in the now. With the aid of props, we rest in poses for five to twenty minutes without strain or pain. You will want to have blocks, bolsters, blankets, and straps, or things you already have at home or work: pillows, couch cushions, and books. We will use all of these things to support you in getting physically comfortable in each pose. You will then hold the pose for an extended period of time.

Dr. Gail Parker, the author of *Restorative Yoga for Ethnic and Race-Based Stress and Trauma*, says,

> *When we practice Restorative Yoga, we are teaching our nervous system how to release contraction and to feel safe coming into deep states of rest that support repair, rejuvenation, and resilience. We are developing a nervous system with a buffer while strengthening our psychological immune system. When we learn to experience our emotional pain and discomfort without contracting around it and reacting to it, and instead just let it move through us, our nervous system becomes regulated, and we become emotionally regulated.* *

I teach, share, and write about restorative yoga because it saved me from a profoundly dysregulated nervous system. Years ago, I overworked, dehydrated, and fatigued myself

---

*Gail Parker, *Restorative Yoga for Ethnic and Race-Based Stress and Trauma* (London: Singing Dragon, 2020), 37.

to the point that I ended up in the hospital with a condition called rhabdomyolysis. My kidneys were near failure, and the emergency room team told me that had I waited another twenty-four hours, I would have been in a far worse condition with lifelong consequences.

And you know what? I almost didn't go to the hospital that morning because I had a big project due at work. I didn't want to bother or worry anyone. Plus, I thought I could just push through the pain and discomfort I was feeling. I even drove myself to the ER despite my husband pleading with me to let him take me. I did not need help. I shouted at him. I was fine!

There was one nurse who took a special interest in me. One evening, she came and sat on my bed and asked, "Sweetheart, why are you in here?"

I responded, "You looked at my chart, right?"

The nurse was unbothered by my rude response and said, "I read all of your charts. I also see you in here reading your lil' yoga books, with your lavender, listening to your 'relaxing' music. Yet, you are still in here for rhabdomyolysis. Something that is so rare and so dangerous. Why? What really landed you in here? Your chart says 'muscles breaking down.' I want you to tell me, if you know, what else is breaking down within you."

I had no words as I looked out the window and held back tears.

Since I couldn't speak, she continued. "We have your physical condition noted, and you will be fine once we get you hydrated and rested, which will take a few days. I need to talk to you about your mind and your heart, though. Seems to me like you've been trying to work yourself to the bone and like you are carrying a whole lot of heavy stuff. Can you put it down?"

She said so much. Finally, she talked to me about the power of rest. She shared her daily and weekly rest practice with me. One that included turning everything off (including her phone) and simply laying down. A practice that she was devoted to despite working twelve- to fourteen-hour shifts, and being a mother, grandmother, wife, and staying active in her community, church, and so much more.

I listened to her sermon (it felt like that) with bated breath. She was telling me a truth that I didn't know I needed to hear.

She didn't have to minister to me on such a personal level, but she did. In doing so, she called me to the altar and held space for me to realize the scary truth: I was afraid to rest. I thought my entire worth was in what I could do and produce for others, even if it meant I worked myself to the point that I collapsed.

She ended our talk by looking deep into my eyes and saying, "Don't you ever forget these words. I live by them. Let them guide you through this and forward. Psalm 46:10: 'Be still and know . . .'"

Be still and know. Be still.
Pause, Rest, Be.

I had already been teaching yoga for a while at that point. Primarily power, hot, and movement/work-out–oriented yoga. That hospitalization showed me what I was teaching and practicing wasn't fully serving me, my students, and the pace of our lives.

My relationship to the power of stillness shifted, and my devotion to rest was conceived in a hospital bed. I prayed a simple prayer, "Lord, give me courage to let go. Let me have faith to trust that I can rest."

It was slow going and required inner reckoning. I didn't just all of a sudden shift to a place of more balance between rest and work. Movement and stillness. Doing and being. I've had to untangle myself from conditioning, guilt, shame, fear of being seen as lazy, and so much more every single day since that fateful moment. I have literally leaned on and been supported by restorative yoga when I felt like my world was crumbling as I navigated endings, liminal space, and beginnings.

My friend and colleague Gina Minyard reminded me, "The Shiva Sutras 2.6 says *gurur upayah*. It can mean that the spiritual teacher (guru) is the means (*upaya*) to enlightenment. It can also be translated to mean that the means (upaya) is the guru. I have always loved that—the practice is the guru."

It hasn't been easy, and I wouldn't take anything for the journey that brought me to one of my greatest teachers, a guru even: restorative yoga.

———

Endings, beginnings, and the space in between are often weighted with emotion, stress, feeling, and discomfort. As we journey through *Pause, Rest, Be*, we will turn toward restorative yoga and rest as a way to be more deeply held to face whatever arises as we do.

Many of us are always holding: holding feelings in, holding children and partners up, holding departments and teams together, or holding aging or sick parents in our hearts and with our hands. Restorative yoga invites us to release and be held. Many of us don't have much practice being held, so this style of yoga that brings us to a place of shapelessness, of being cradled, can lead us to feel some emotional vulnerability and even discomfort. When this happens, feel. Stay with the breath and allow it to pass.

Pause, Rest, Be is a call into the universal classroom of right now. An invitation to reflect on our individual and collective lives, how our past informs the present, and how to carry our best heart and wisdom forward in thoughts, actions, and deeds. This requires us to put down much of what we've been carrying, clinging, and holding on to. To listen for a new way within the quiet of our hearts. To pose less and practice more presence through stillness and rest. To get closer to the ground, to bow at the feet of our Beloved Teacher. That Beloved Teacher I am speaking of is a practice rooted in stillness: restorative yoga.

To begin your journey, you will want to have:

- A journal and something to write with. I am sure inner knowing will emerge as you journey through this book.
- Pillows, blankets, and bolsters—things that will allow you to create a comfortable and soft place to land, rest,

and practice a restorative pose before or after reading a
chapter.

- If you have the ability to designate a special place or
corner in your home to be your place to be with *Pause,
Rest, Be*, carve out that space. Leave your book, journal,
and props there. Bless that space as you start.

With so much suddenly shifting, now we are ready to go deeper.
Alone and together.

Let us begin with the end.

PART ONE

Endings

When faced with an ending, an all-of-a-sudden ending, what do you do? What can we do when what we once knew and believed to be infallible begins to crumble before our eyes? When our inner and outer worlds are writhing in unexpected and prolonged pain? When the reckoning of ages has come slowly and then all at once?

We can turn away. We can pretend that the communal death bed isn't overflowing. We can turn and try to run backward toward a place that no longer exists.

A place that was a facade to begin with.

We can numb ourselves with overconsumption of all things good and not so good.

We can close our eyes and tightly squeeze them shut.

We can turn our backs on reality and then what?

None of that stops what is coming. It only renders us completely unprepared when an end arrives.

Beloveds, there are so many endings crashing down at once. Can we sit alone and feel the magnitude of all of this? Then, can we sit together and strengthen our breath? Where my inhale is strong and yours is weak, can you be my exhale? Will you drum against your heart with me and call on everything that is sacred, holy, and timeless to have mercy on us all?

Let's begin with the end.

Corpse Pose | Savasana

A Pose for Endings

I remember the first yoga class I ever took. It was hot; it was sweaty. We worked and worked. We pushed and pushed. We tried and tried. At the end of the pose, we came to the ground and were instructed to simply lie flat and close our eyes. The teacher called this pose *Savasana*. He said it translated to "Corpse Pose." A place where we die, we end, a place that promised rebirth and a new beginning. He also said it was the most important pose, or asana, in all of yoga. I was completely perplexed. I don't remember much of what he said after that point because I couldn't stop thinking about how it was possible to twist, turn, bend, and contort my body, to fight with my muscles and bones to make the "just right shape" only to be told by my teacher that "laying on the ground and being still" is the most important thing you can do.

As I lay there turning this idea over in my mind, I did hear one final perplexing thing. He said, "Savasana is also likely the most difficult pose you will encounter." After class, I hurriedly packed all of my things and ran up to my teacher. Exasperated, I asked, "But why is Savasana so important? I mean, we aren't even doing anything in that pose. Nothing is happening." He smiled and said, "Keep practicing and come to understand it for yourself." That was seventeen years ago.

Descriptions of Savasana as an asana date back to the *Hatha Yoga Pradipika*, a fifteenth-century text in which we find many of the earliest references to the yoga poses that are still practiced today. It is the only pose among all the asanas that is included in every sequence, a hint to its importance. I didn't know about the Hatha Yoga Pradipika in my earliest yoga days, and even if I had,

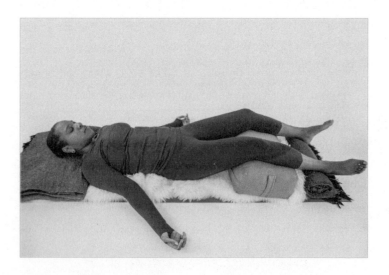

I still would have been confused by the "non-doing" postures as I'd come to associate yoga with movement and doing. Despite making the connection that it is, in fact, the one pose included in every class, it took years for me to become curious enough to return to my first teacher's words about Savasana: "It's the most important . . . It's challenging." It was then that I actually became a student of this posture and journeyed into the heart of this way of ending.

After a much longed-for and hoped-for pregnancy ended in a painful miscarriage, I didn't know what to do with myself or my body. I remember going to a class, telling the teacher I was in pain, and her suggesting that I lie down and breathe. Savasana. I knew I couldn't physically practice, and I also knew I needed to be in a room with other people. I didn't want to be alone. I didn't move one muscle, yet the first moments in Savasana were a mental and emotional fight. I wanted to move. I wanted to do something. I needed to fix it. Fix me. Fix my body. Fix the part I perceived was so broken that I couldn't even hold a pregnancy, a hope, a dream.

And then it happened—my body stopped gripping. I cried. I surrendered to the earth beneath me. I allowed myself to feel the end, the end of that excitement, the end of that expectation, the end of that pregnancy, the end of the part of me who innocently longed to be a mother and wanted it all to be so easy.

5

Savasana both challenged me and held space for my endings that day. Savasana became one of my Beloved Teachers.

———

Ultimately, I have come to understand Savasana as the practice of death, and every ending, big or small, is some kind of death. In Savasana, we practice the death of the ego, death of grasping, and death of all aversion to reality as it is. In Savasana, we practice recognizing that *for now*, there's nothing left to do. I've also learned that when we are particularly activated with fear, worry, or anxiety related to endings, it's best that we cocoon and support ourselves in Savasana instead of simply lying down. In that way, we create a place to be held, cradled, and supported through and in this most potent and powerful pose and place. This ending. Savasana.

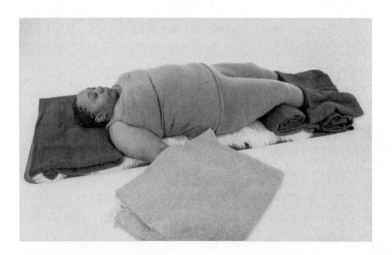

What You Need to Practice

A yoga mat, 6–8 blankets, one bolster or couch cushion, cozy socks, *Pause, Rest, Be*, a journal, and something to write with.

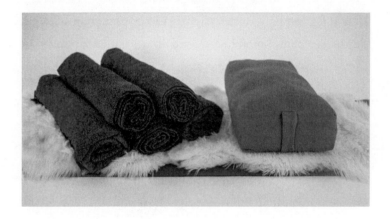

How to Set Up

TIME: 5–15 minutes

Create a landing place. Put down a yoga mat and layer on two blankets folded in half on top of your mat. This gives you a soft place to land. Then lie down. Place a rolled blanket or bolster under your knees to encourage the thighbones to drop deeper into your pelvis, relieving tension in the iliopsoas. The pelvis will rest more heavily against the ground because of this. If you would like to feel more tucked in, wrap a blanket around your ankles. Place a folded blanket over your belly to release tension and weigh the hips down even more. Place blankets under your arms and hands so that they aren't touching the floor. Rest your arms by your sides, palms facing down.

If your upper back and shoulders are rolled toward your heart and don't rest easily on the floor, place a folded blanket or towel underneath your head, neck, and tips of your shoulders so you feel support all the way up the torso to your neck and head. Your chin should be perpendicular to the floor and your throat should feel open and at ease. Cover your entire body with a blanket or two if you would like.

Once You Are in It

Begin by keeping your eyes open and noticing how your body feels. Scan your body from the top of your head to the tips of your toes, from the tips of your toes to the top of your head. Do this 3–5 times, allowing yourself to notice what you feel and where you feel it. If you are feeling worried or agitated, I invite you to keep your eyes open for the duration of the posture or just a little while longer. Sometimes, immediately closing our eyes takes us on a trip to Worry Land if we are already a little turnt up. If you keep your eyes open, let them be soft and focused on one place. If you are ready to drop in, close your eyes. Either way, with each exhalation, allow the earth beneath you to fully hold each part of your body. Once you feel completely connected to the ground, sense that whatever is in your mind can also be held by the earth, and give it to her. Once you feel more space between each thought, take your awareness to the center of your chest. Feel and notice. If something is weighing on your heart, know that the earth can hold that as well. Exhale deeply and give your heart's burdens to the earth. With awareness at your own heart, offer up an intention or prayer for courage and support with whatever endings you are facing. Rest your awareness and intention on the waves of your breath. Stay in the pose for 5–15 minutes. When coming out, bend your knees, roll onto your right side, and rest in a fetal-like position.

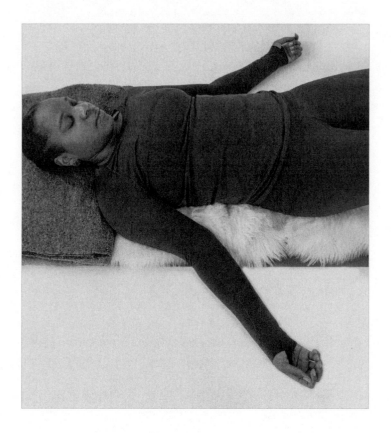

After the Pose

We roll from Savasana to the fetal position. Journal or draw for 2–3 minutes. Reconnect to your intention or prayer. Hold *Pause, Rest, Be* at your heart. Open to a page. Allow the message you need for support through an ending to find you.

As we slowly move out of Savasana, we intentionally return and explore our body, heart, and mind as though they are new because, after Savasana, they are. This reminds us that every ending transforms into a beginning at some point.

Considerations

If you have a hard time settling in or being still, do one of the following before you rest:

1. Turn on your favorite song with drums and bass tones in it and dance.
2. Shake. Yes, shake your body. Start by shaking your feet, then swirling your hips. Next, shake your hands. Shake your whole body.
3. Feel into the place in your body that is least settled or able to be still. Ask that place how it needs to move. Move the way it needs you to for 5–10 minutes.

I

Ain't No Turning 'Round

Six months is not long unless the world is turned upside down. Then, six months is a lifetime.

And in that lifetime, you walk over hot coals of rage while stumbling through despair and falling over the edge of fear. You land beyond that edge and pray at the altar of uncertainty. You put down some of what you've been carrying. You put down things like the need to control, "what it looks like" and attachment to "there must be one answer" because you realize how long the road you must walk is. Within that realization, you sense that over the course of walking, any answers you think you have will transform into more questions along the way.

You kneel down until beautiful scars replace your knees.

When you get up, you walk differently. Because, well . . . after all of that, you can never be the same.

You do not look behind you. You do not look ahead of you.

The only thing to see is this place where you have fallen down, bowed, and finally stood up from.

And in the lifetime of six months, you become the kind of wise that your elders said comes with living. And you realize that what they were really talking about is "living through" so many endings that you have no choice but to let go and grow. Maya Angelou's final message on Twitter said,

> *Listen to yourself, and in that quietude, you might hear the voice of God.*

Even now, may the wisdom of these words echo in our hearts and guide our decisions, choices, affirmations, and boundaries.

The road you are walking is not linear. It is long, has some ruts, and is unpaved. It may feel like an obstacle, and it is also a way.

It is a way home.

What obstacle are you facing on your personal road? One that may look like an end? Are you willing to consider that it may be the way or a beginning? It's okay if the answer is no today. One day, it may be yes.

2

In Destruction, Create Refuge

I source wisdom from many places. Early in the pandemic of 2020 and one day while talking to my mama about all that was shifting, being revealed, ending, disappearing, and showing she got really quiet.

Then she said, "As I continue to stay close to home, be still, and look at what's all going on in the world, I've been thinking how everybody thought Noah was crazy, gathering up things and building that ark. They thought he was out of his mind 'til it started to rain. Daughter, the ark is a place of inner refuge and shelter. Stay close to the ark 'cause the rain ain't even started yet. You stay close to the ark all the way through and 'til the end."

For me, the story of Noah's ark is one of creation, existence, and destruction.

That holy cycle is one that we are always in and one that is more pronounced and accelerated over the last few months and years.

For me, building the ark means I fortify myself daily through rest, writing, meaningfully connecting to the community, and tending to my resources and time with intention.

Staying close to the ark means I acknowledge when something big is shifting either in the collective that affects my personal life or in my personal life that impacts how I see, experience, and engage with the collective.

Collective change is upon us all, and it is deeply personal.

The illusion that we will make it through the flooding without getting wet—I see that ending too, and the dawning reality is not pretty. It is so real, and in that way, it contains its own beauty.

There are more rains ahead. Yesterday has ended. Beloved, you will need refuge. Build your ark.

Take a moment to sit and breathe into the moment you are in. Feel your breath take refuge in your body while also providing your body refuge. Bring to mind someone or something that brings you a sense of refuge or being held. For a few breaths, hold the image of that person or thing in your mind. Then let the image go and allow yourself to be within the essence they provide. Refuge.

3

Why Rush the End?

Let's say today is the last day of the world as you know it. Are you going to multitask your way through it? Giving nothing and no one full, devoted attention—not even yourself?

Are you going to allow "doing the most" to steal your joy and intimacy?

You know that feeling. Talking to someone on the phone, online, or even in person, you sense a kind of vacancy. Like they are "there" and gone at the same time. The connection has ended before it even starts because they aren't paying attention. We might want to take it personally and internalize their lack of attention to us as evidence that we don't deserve undivided presence. Yet, it's not personal. It's a pattern. One that so many of us act out over and over even with ourselves.

If we don't know how to be with ourselves without distractions and multitasking, how can we be with anyone else?

We also know the feeling. Talking to someone—whether in person, on the phone, or online—and they are completely there. Fully present. Something in us wakes up. We feel seen. Heard. Our breath deepens and becomes fuller. We fall in love with the moment and person in front of us.

If this day, hour, and minute were the end of the world as I know it, I would:

> Drink a cup of tea with my love and silently watch his eyes.
> I'd play cars and trucks with my son and laugh at the top of my lungs about nothing in particular.
> I'd wear my cutest dress. Listen to a song until I could trace the rhythm to my heartbeat, and slow dance with myself.
> I'd read one single paragraph in a whole book, word by word by word. Just one paragraph though, out loud to my family so that we could commit the words to memory together.
> Or perhaps, I'd sit alone and feel the weight of my body against the ground and allow myself to be completely touched by the earth.

I'd do all of the things that look like I am doing nothing in our fast-paced culture, like simply doing one thing at a time.

I'd remember just how rich and full *nothing* or *one thing at a time* can be.

Release yourself from the jaws of multitasking and divided attention.

Savor. Don't wait. Savor now.

Eat your next meal slow, steady, with devotion. Like it's your last meal in that particular place and time. The simple truth is . . . well, it always actually is.

4

Feeling Our Way Through

Joy is an act of rebellion. And so is allowing ourselves to feel our grief.

We can only access as much joy as we have the capacity to feel our sorrow, our pain, our losses, and what hurts our hearts.

Feeling.

Feeling is a profound act of rebellion when you've been conditioned to stuff everything in. Overwork and grind it away. Pretend it away. Bypass it away. Joke it away. Pray it away. Fuss and fight it away.

Do anything, just Get. It. Away. Those feelings!

As I feel my way through the grief of the last few years and unacknowledged sorrows of days gone by, I see clearly. Joy is, in fact, what we all come from. Living and feeling my way through *it all* expands my ability to return to it—joy. To enter the place where joy resides. To embrace it and be held by it once I get there. To allow the door to the sanctuary of joy to oscillate—as it naturally does—versus cling to the knob of it because I fear the feelings that exist outside of the door of joy.

Can you fully experience the depth of joy if you can't face your suffering and pain in a real way?

If you are going to make it through, *this now*, you have to feel. Acknowledge your feelings. Dance with them. Shake with them. Create with them. Sit with them. Rock with them. Cry with them. Shout with them. Moan with them. Tell ourselves, friends, therapists, pastors, and lovers the truth about them.

Feeling is a profound act of rebellion.

Feel as an act of reclamation of your wholeness. Feel as an act of faith. Feel as a way to honor your heart.

No matter your spiritual or religious background, may you find solace in these words: "Weeping may endure for the night. Joy will come in the morning" (Psalms 30:5).

Even when that morning feels far away.

Even when that morning feels far away.

Say this to yourself and mean it: Today, I allow myself to feel my feelings: messy, loud, curled up in a ball, hands extended in delight, lips curled in sweetness, fires of rage, rivers of tears—the range of feeling. Today, I allow myself to feel. Then, allow yourself a pause, some space, and time to do just that.

5

Listen Closely

What voice is the most reliable? Who is there to trust? Every other report is conflicting.

People are fighting on the internet, in the streets, in their houses, and in the hospitals. Fighting for their lives.

Many are fighting for a return to a world that no longer exists. A world that is a flickering memory.

People are getting sick. People are healing. From viruses and a multitude of pain they didn't have time to name until now. And others are filling up all of the time to avoid feeling anything other than the tapping beneath their fingers as they work and work and work.

She won't stay inside. He won't leave the house. She's frozen in fear. He's moved over his edge.

But, "Whose report will you believe?"

Whose voice is the loudest in your ear? What message is on repeat in your head? Is it your voice or someone else's? Is it your Divine or something else?

Lean into the practices, rituals, and prayers that keep you close to your intuition. To pure wisdom and the spirit of discernment.

Believe the report that arrives when you tune in.

Believe the report that arrives when you tune in from within.

⌒

> *Take a moment to pause. Either sit down or place your feet on the ground. Connect to your breath and listen. This is one simple and profound way to tune in. What do you notice? What do you hear from within when you listen closely?*

6

It's Dark. Rest. Then Keep Going.

As a teacher and mentor, I know that I can't be responsible for leading anyone deeper than I've gone. To stay within integrity and alignment, I have to be honest when I've walked with a student or mentee as far as I can go with them.

As a student, I have come to many dark edges and had teachers who reminded me where I hid my light when I forgot that it was inside of me.

I've also come to wild and strange places. Just as I was about to enter the darkest part, I received the message, "That path ahead is for you to go without me."

"Without me" doesn't mean no presence.

Some people / teachers know they can't go with us. Those teachers hold vigil. They stay at the base camp and tend to the fire that we'll need when we make it home. They pray for us on our journeys, and they release us to our destinies.

Sometimes the teacher is a single person. Sometimes the teacher is our mama or papa. Sometimes the teacher is our partner or even our child. Sometimes the teacher is a whole community holding space for us, even as they let us go to become who we were born to be.

The map for our most sacred expedition is often only revealed when we are brave enough to step into the unknown, be guided by the light in our heart, the rhythm of our own feet, and the compass of our breath.

At the darkest turn, we may think we are alone. Remember.

Remember someone's tending the fire and trusting you'll make it through.

Broken. Undone. Shifted. Transformed. Yet through.

It is dark in some patches of the journey. Keep going.

You are healing.

You will return.

Reflect and remember a time when you physically walked alone yet knew you were being guided and supported by forces, seen and unseen. What did that feel like in your body and heart? Pause. Remember. Say thank you.

7

Turbulent Landings

Waiting for someone you love to die is hovering ten thousand feet in the air, frozen yet trembling. Is a crash coming?

It is the fear of falling to sleep because you don't want to miss the last five hundred breaths they take.

It is waking up to see the sun yet stumbling through days in darkness. It is hearing laughter and wishing today was as easy as that sound. It is stinging cold on the hottest day of the year.

You look at the phone when it rings and you decide that if you don't answer, you don't have to talk about "comfort" care or how many hours there may be left of what the nurse said is "natural life."

If you have ever watched someone about to leave their body, you know that God isn't always beautiful, and, without a doubt, she's real. You know sometimes there is a fight. You know there is no winning or losing. There simply is.

Watching my grandmother watch her firstborn—my dad—die, I learned that mamas never stop seeing the innocence of their baby and always remember the complete joy and pain of their child's first breath.

If you've ever watched and waited for someone you love to die, you know your whole world changes like the air in the room. In some places, it thins so they can pass through the veil to the next world. In other places, it thickens to hold all the love and memories in.

You know that the spaces outside of the waiting room feel like betrayal. The way everyone else's time seems to move on while you watch for it to stop in a forever kind of way.

You know that every prayer is heard and ain't always answered in ways we can understand. You know that in the rawest of moments, prayer is a covering for your heart. You know that when everything is pulled apart at the seams, prayer is the thread that holds the smallest part of us together.

You know what it is to retrace a lifetime of memories, only to realize there are too many gaps and no way to fill them in. You hold on to faith that those places will indeed be where the light streams through.

You know that sometimes silence is a loud and deafening sound.

After days and nights of waiting and watching, when Charles Ramsey—my dad—left his body, I remember trying to steady my feet on the ground and root down, yet feeling caught ten thousand and then nine thousand and then eight thousand feet in the air, waiting to crash.

It gets turbulent and rocky. You may need to close the window and your eyes on this ride because there is nothing to see out there.

After losing someone you love, you will eventually land. You land with your feet and heart deeper in the earth.

We land closer to all living things and everything that has breath. We land closer to the hem of God's torn yet regal garment. Braver in the face of the grit, stuff, compost within us all.

⁓

Honor someone you have loved and lost by listening to a song that reminds you of them. Move or dance to the song, or perhaps you simply rest.

8

Come by Here

I know this is true. When we call, God comes.

Come by here, my lord, come by here. Come by yuh, my lord.
*Come by yuh. Kumbaya, Kumbaya.**

During my sixty-ish hours of labor with my son, I consulted
all of my logical, rational book knowledge. I clung to the plan
I made even though my first encounter with a real contraction
devoured that plan and spat it in my face. I tensed against every
wave for hours and thought that if I could just get it together
and control my body, I could control my labor.

Come by here, my lord, come by here. Come by yuh, come by
yuh. Kumbaya, Kumbaya.

---

*African American spiritual, unknown origin.

In the literal fifty-sixth hour. Exhausted. Weary and after looking for an escape, only to realize that the only way out is through. In that fifty-sixth hour, I turned to my doula. I turned to my husband. I turned to my nurse and midwife. I said, "I need Jesus to come by here. I need Oshun. I need Yemaya. I need every elevated Ancestral mother and grandmother I have. I need all of them to come by here."

My doula began to sing. "Come by here, come by here. Come by yuh, come by yuh. Kumbaya, Kumbaya." She added names and mamas as she sang. I called, and they came.

It was the most sacred roll call of my life, and I felt the presence of everything holy as each name called entered.

Only after I had surrendered my plans, will, ego, and ideas of how it ought to be and called out to The Divine did my baby turn and drop down. The rest of the journey was glorious and ecstatic.

I could have called at any time, yet for me, it took hours (equivalent to months in labor—ha!) to let go and accept *this*. This is how it is.

Right now, you may be in a long labor and at the fifty-sixth hour—a time of immense destruction and creation. Birth.

May you have the strength to surrender and call.
Dear God, come by yuh, come by yuh. Stop by our hearts.

Kumbaya, Kumbaya. Enter our minds.

Come by here, come by here. Visit this place, and stay awhile.

We need to see you. We need to hear a word from you.

Come by here.

⌇

Write a prayer for yourself and humanity. Let it flow from your heart. Speak it out loud. Trust you are heard. You are felt.

9

Missing Stars

The next time we sing and call in Ancestors.

The next time we pour libations, we will say her name.

And she will come. Wearing new robes, held together with words written by Audre, June, Lucille, Maya, and Ntozake to welcome her into the next world.

And she will say something like, "Something that is loved is never lost."*

And she will stand at the edge of our circle and call us into the center, one by one. She will listen deeply as we excavate our stories from our souls. There will be wailing and laughter. There will be cussing and prayers. There will be slurs and

---

*Toni Morrison, *Beloved* (New York: Vintage, 1987), 234.

exquisite enunciation. There will be silence and shouting in our testimonies and telling.

She will gather all of it within her majestic dress and spread it across the sky when she flies back.

She is freer now. We've inherited her relentlessness, love, and devotion to the humanity of all beings and Black folks. I've inherited a deeper sense of responsibility to tell my story.

She went to rest, yes. And in a little while, she will come when we call. In our memory, in our hearts, in our words yet to be written, Great Mother, Writer, Warrior, Truth-Teller Toni Morrison lives.

There are people who elevate the human collective and consciousness, and when they leave this earth, we feel it. Name a "star" who has transitioned that inspired and affected your life. How did they affect your life? Why? Through their end, may they encourage you to begin to follow your true North Star.

10

Ending a Legacy of Fear

The day I found out that I was having a baby boy, I cried.

I turned away from the ultrasound screen and a solid stream of tears flowed. The tech said, "Sweetie, you don't want to see?"

I couldn't speak. It wasn't that. I absolutely did want to see. But I turned my back to the image on the screen and wondered *when*.

When would my Black baby boy stop being a baby to the world?
When would my Black boy child stop being a child in the face of institutions?
When did Tamir Rice stop being a child to the officer who killed him?
When did Trayvon Martin stop being a youth to the brute who killed him?
When did their lives stop mattering to people?

I cried because we live in a world where Black men and women are filmed being shot in the back, kneeled on, and choked to death by folk who are supposed to "serve and protect" and the first question many ask is, *"Well . . .* what did *they* do?" *They* being the person who is no longer breathing.

I cried because I've been a public and private school teacher, and I've seen how office referrals for little Black boys read like criminal reports even when it's behavior that other boys get deemed as "just being a kid," and I know that this discrepancy reflects one that is indicative of a much greater one within our criminal justice system within the United States.

I cried because I'm sick of the propaganda stations called "news" that just can't get enough of "documenting" "Black-on-Black" crime when we know white-collar crime is destroying our world—and often just considered business as usual.

Does anyone else not see the connection between the images we are "fed" about groups of people and how it shapes and forms our ideas about who we assume people are? *But I digress* . . .

I wondered when someone will follow my Black son through a store, hug their purse closer to them when he walks by, skip the elevator he is on, or call a cop because he "looks suspicious" or "fits a description." These are everyday experiences for me and even more so for my husband in public places.

I cried. Then I exhaled and smiled.

Even in all of that, I felt an overwhelming sense of protection and possibility for and from my boy as I do in his father's arms and presence.

My son is an incredible human.

We raise him with joy, pride, love, and freedom. We challenge and we raise him to challenge any perceptions of who he ought to be. By the time both my husband and I were six years old we had learned how to walk through the world and see from all sides at all times in order to perceive threats and try to protect our small Black bodies. As we teach our son to remain aware, we grapple with how to release and no longer transmit the fear we have lived with and contorted our being around.

The day I found out I was bringing a Black son into this world, I cried, realizing it is a calling and the honor of a lifetime. Then I turned my gaze back to where my baby boy wiggled, stretched, and thrived on the screen. I promised him that we will take up room. We will not shrink ourselves for someone else's comfort. We will keep moving forward. We will not forget where we come from. We will live and not be stifled. I promised him that we will grow and live in courage. Loving ourselves fully is one way we live in that courage.

It takes courage to try and understand a reality that directly challenges and/or contradicts our own. Recall a conversation or moment when you felt confronted by someone else's story, experience, or truth. Can you revisit that experience and "put on" new ears? Recall and simply listen. What can you hear when you listen beyond your singular perspective?

11

Down by the Riverside

The gentle is powerful.

I am looking at a river flow—a steady, slow stream. There are heavy rocks anchored beneath the pulsing river. I lean forward to sense the depth and touch the movement of this moment. Up close, I see the rocks worn, clearly affected—transformed even—by the ambling, unhurried dance of water passing eternity after eternity over them.

I look to the river to teach me a way to live, exist, and be.

River speaks to me in whispers and slow rhymes. River says, "Watch me. I am unhurried, and I have been for millions of years. I know my rhythm and the very drumbeat of life. I am soft and fluid, yet I change everything I touch. I am changed by everything that touches me. I resist nothing. Most years, I am gentle."

Here I am. Down by the riverside. So, so much has ended. I have, we all have been changed.

I offer my endings to the river. I offer our collective endings to the river.

I stand here being washed over. Yet, fully participating in the shift. As I am cleansed, I am also worn.

For tomorrow, I carry both the wisdom of the river and the soul of the rock in my heart.

Honestly, I am afraid. Truthfully, I am still brave.

I know one thing for sure: there ain't no turnin' round.

Imagine you are sitting before an ancient river. Listen, imagine you can hear the river song. Vision, see the water flow over rocks. Feel a breeze touch your hands and heart. Taste the cool freshness of the air on your lips. What ending would you like to offer to the river? Turn your palms up. Reach your hands forward. Offer something to the river. Do this as many times as you need to. May you be free and lighter as you make this offering and face this end.

A Prayer for Endings

God of endings,

Even as we face uncertainty, we thank you for walking with us across the river of time. Where we believe all is lost and everything is over, show us how the obstacle is our way. We trust that the endings we face will not end us. We know that some endings signify a much-needed change has come. As humans, we want so terribly to hold on, even when we have prayed for a shift and it arrives at our door. Help us to turn the knob, cross the threshold, and finally close the door on the places that can no longer serve us. Help us to let go and surrender to the dissolution that many endings bring.

If we must fall apart, let the shattering reveal the contents of our hearts, the wisdom that resides there. When we meet endings that break us, let the crevice that opens within point us toward our souls' expansion or at least a ray of hope. When we believe our story is complete and done, be the author of our courage, faith, and truth. May we continue. Hold us and our futures through it all. Be an everlasting arm that we can rest upon and a place for us to restore. Do not let us forget that endings are often brave beginnings dressed in the scariest costume.

PART TWO

Liminal Space

Space in between Endings and Beginnings

What about when now is not an ending or a beginning? If both places are uncomfortable and uncertain, the space in between can feel like total annihilation. Like falling into a canyon: wide, deep, empty, and full. Yet, it can feel like a sliver and easy to miss if we bypass or rush through it—the liminal.

Carols of light and darkness gather and sing in this place. Not songs of grief or joy. Ecstasy or pain. Love or hate. Songs with more silence than words. Songs that pause to listen inward for tears, laughter, fear, bewilderment, despair, longing to determine if the next pulsation will be quiet or full of sound.

When now is not an end or a beginning, it is the middle of a road. This place is not to be confused with the half point because our destination is concealed, and we don't know how far we have come or how far we have to go. The modes of travel that we have depended on are no longer reliable. Normalcy is suspended. We have been hurled into space with no promise of the way we will return or if returning is even possible.

Once we've entered this portal that exists between "no longer" and "not yet," the liminal space, an initiation is underway. This is a veiled place where the world we thought we knew vanishes, and there is nothing on the horizon because the horizon has been swallowed by time. Hidden. Mysterious. Unknown of cosmic proportions.

Like caterpillars making their way toward their cocoon, we have crawled our way through endings. Yet it is unclear what we are becoming.

Caterpillars must enter a liminal space to grow their wings. In that space, they literally dissolve into goop. In that soup of slime, there are cells that will become the magnificent thing that kisses flowers in bloom—a butterfly. Those cells are called "imaginal cells." The mystery of imaginal cells is that they are not assigned to anything in advance. They may become an eye, a wing, or an antenna. What every single cell will become cannot be determined within the caterpillar. It must disintegrate first.

It must completely break down and become unrecognizable to itself and the world.

Between endings and beginnings, our old self vanishes.

Our vision is often challenged in liminal spaces. It is where we must learn how to see in the dark. Our eyes have to adjust to the radiance within our shadows and the tenebrosity that dwells in our light.

Here we are at a departure and arrival point. Exhaustedly realizing that what worked in the past will not work here in this environment. It's messy, and we may cry a lot. Each tear is an imaginal cell. We may endlessly sigh. Each breath is an imaginal cell. We may writhe, rage, moan, and kick about. Each movement unleashes an imaginal cell. We may crouch in the corner, afraid to move. We will most definitely lie on our sides, curl into ourselves, and call on all that is sacred to see us through. Rest and stillness allow the imaginal cells to slowly form into the signposts, paths, and vessels that point us forward.

Or perhaps we are the imaginal cell within the great organism of humanity. We have been deconstructed in order to put ourselves back together in a way that not only heals us but also our families, community, and world.

Either way, liminal space holds imaginal cells. Without it, there are no beginnings. No metamorphosis or transformation. Without it, we have no wings to rise.

Beloved, as we drop beneath the surface of what is known, we enter a place of possibility. A place where the one thing I am sure of is this: I do not know what this part of the path holds. I do know that we are held.

Everything and nothing exists here.

Side-Lying Pose | Parsva Savasana

A Pose for the Space In Between

Her eyes were piercing, dark, yet they glowed with a menacing and destructive fire as she peered down at me, blew her whistle in my face, cackled, and then referenced the 1992 movie. Though she was right in my face, she yelled loud enough for the entire gym of girls to hear. "You say white men can't jump? Huh! Well, from the looks of your god-awful-freaking-terrible shooting, looks like little Black girls can't jump! Get off my court with that streetball!"

The Women's National Basketball Association was still a few years away, but up until that point, I dreamed of basketball being a part of my future. If you asked me who I was in middle school, I would have said two things: I'm a nerd. I'm a baller.

In a place like middle school, those two identities often present a kind of paradox. I was quirky and lacked the courage and confidence to try out for the official school team until eighth grade, when I realized it's now or never, at least for middle school.

So that day, on that court, I was working my hardest and bringing all of the braveheartedness, precision, skill, and love of the game that I had to basketball tryouts. As one of two Black girls going out for a team that was always white in a school that was 95 percent white, I was beyond nervous. My every move was judged and measured. My mistakes were announcements that I wasn't just a failure; my race was. I remember missing one jump shot. Then another. Then she, the well-respected, grown white woman coach, was in my face, yelling at me with such joy and confirmation, "Looks like little Black girls can't jump! Get off my court with that streetball!"

The ball no longer dribbled and pulsed. My heart stopped as her words shot through my veins.

I held myself together and walked off the court.

When I made it to the locker room, I fell to the ground, landed on my side, and stayed in that position alone for some time. Too stunned to cry. Too afraid to make any sound, lest I'd be the raging Black girl. Too tired to move. I tried to catch my breath even as I felt a part of me die.

After that day, I didn't call myself a baller anymore. It was lost to me as I entered a void-like space in relation to that aspect of my identity. That painful experience abruptly pushed me from what I thought was a promising beginning to an ending, and then to an undefined space before I could begin again.

Years later, and in a restorative yoga immersion specifically designed to support Black women and Women of Color with race-based stress and trauma, led by Dr. Gail Parker, I found my way back into that pose that I'd intuitively gone to that day in the gym: Side-Lying Pose. This time, I hadn't run from a lady with blazing racism roaring from her eyes. This time, I didn't collapse down into the pose. With agency, I had walked into a room that felt like a brave space. I'd summoned my courage to face whatever would emerge in such a place. I'd carefully set myself up with blankets and bolsters. I had settled and nestled myself into a side-lying position.

———

Side-Lying Pose is a pose in between facing upright and facing down. It is a pose that cradles us as we approach the edge of before and after. With a masterful, kind, and compassionate teacher, resting in that pose is where I had the audacity to reenter the court. As I rested in the pose, I listened to the rise and fall of my breath. I heard a ball bounce in the distance. I did not know if that sound was merely in my head or outside of the room. My body began to contract. I tried desperately to hold on. The support of the props beneath and around me reminded me I didn't have to. *Keep breathing. Keep breathing.* This became my mantra. That refrain, coupled with breath and the length of time we stayed in the pose, finally loosened my grip. The bolster between my knees and ankles became my leg.

Behind my closed eyes, I began to see the court. The fire in that coach's eyes. The fallout and destruction from those flames. My head nestled against the blanket as I remembered something else: that day I held my head high as I left that particularly wretched court. I also recounted something else: the love I had for the essence of the sport. As I breathed and rested, that love sat eye to eye, knee to knee, and heart to heart with the hate I experienced that day during tryouts. Reentering the void, that place between face down or face up, returned me to a place of possibility. I emerged from that safe cradle of resting inside a side-lying position, knowing it was part of my journey to reclaim this piece of my identity: baller.

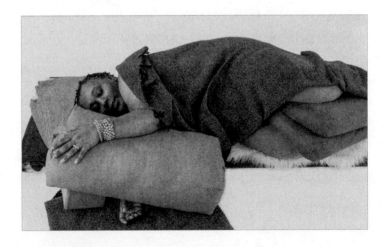

―――――

Parsva translates to "side" or "plank." We have learned and know that *savasana* means "corpse." In more active styles of yoga, we come into Side-Lying Pose, or Parsva Savasana, when we are leaving our time in Savasana and before we sit up, bow, and enter the next part of our day or evening. In movement-oriented classes, we don't usually linger in this pose, and still, the spaciousness of it is usually the moment where something unexpected is revealed. It's the moment in class when I most readily realize what I have released, gained, or more deeply accessed in the entire yoga session. At least, that has been my experience of even just 30–60 seconds of resting on my side.

Parsva Savasana is also referred to as the fetal position. In a spontaneous or organic fetal position, the back is curved, the limbs bent and drawn in toward the midline. The head is tucked toward the heart. The various names of this shape point to the power of it. It is both death and birth. It is also neither.

―――――

In March 2013, my mother suffered a heart attack that her surgeon said he hadn't seen anyone else with the level of blockage survive. She had walked around for days feeling like something just wasn't quite right, alternating between dizziness and buzzy energy—shortness of breath and a rapid pulse. What began as a slow ache in her left arm progressed into a searing pain by day three. Still believing that it was "no big deal," a family member drove her to the hospital instead of her taking an ambulance. On the way there, she instinctively rolled to one side and curled up. By the time she ended up in the emergency room, she said she was not here, not in her body. She said the place she inhabited during that time looked like equal parts pure darkness and blinding light.

What she remembers from that day is that she was in a place that she describes as "like a void." She said, "I could see my body and life as an intimate witness, but I couldn't hear anything for a while. Not even my own breath." She says one voice and sound did finally emerge within that liminal space that she hovered in. *Grandma. Grandma. Grandma.* She heard someone saying, "Grandma." And then the darkness dissolved into light. First, shimmering and streaming particles. Then the fluorescent lights of the hospital room. She inhaled and felt her body. She was alive.

One year later, almost at the exact time and on the day of my mother's heart attack, my niece was born. I don't share this story to even begin to pontificate where we go from here or whether we can will ourselves back into our body when we are leaving this earth plane. I share it because it holds the essence of liminality within it—death and rebirth. I share it because it shows us that there is always something, be it root, seed, or blossom, waiting to be revealed in that space. I share it because my mother somehow just knew to turn inward. I share it because it is evidence to me of the amazing grace that meets us within our most disorienting, terrifying, and anguished places.

It is amazing grace that moves us toward our hearts' center and the silence that resides there so that we can hear beyond the noise we accumulate in our lives. It is amazing grace that finds us when we have spun ourselves in circles, tried to walk everyone else's path, and ultimately become lost. It is amazing grace that recalibrates our eyes so that we can see. I have experienced so much of that amazing grace in this side-lying posture. The grace of falling apart in a cold locker room and being held. The grace of returning to that place in my heart and reclaiming a cherished part of my identity. The grace of my beloved mother accessing a future memory and it calling her back into the present.

———

If you find yourself at the edge of both night and day, hovering at the rim of complete destruction and creation, rest here. If you are treading along the nebulous margin of no longer and not yet, rest here. If you don't quite know how or why it ended, rest here. If you doubt that you will ever have the will, courage, or desire to begin again, rest here. Rest here on your side. Allow amazing grace to enter.

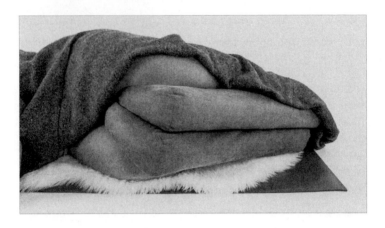

What You Need to Practice

A yoga mat, six to eight blankets, two bolsters or a couch cushion, one pillow, cozy socks, *Pause, Rest, Be*, a journal, and something to write with.

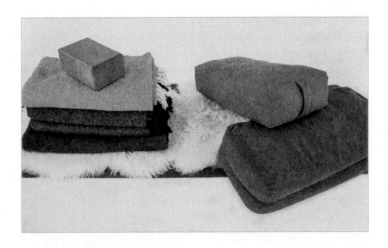

How to Set Up

TIME: 10–15 minutes

Create a landing place. Put down a yoga mat and layer on two blankets folded in half on top of your mat. This gives you a soft place to land. Fold at least two blankets into pillows. Have all props close by.

Choose your favorite side and lie down with your head and neck resting on one or two of the pillows you created. Make sure that your neck is fully supported and not higher or lower than the rest of your spine.

Check in with your shoulders to ensure that they are stacked and parallel to one another. In other words, one shoulder is not in front of the other.

Make sure that your hips are level as well. Then place one of the bolsters, pillows, or couch cushions between your knees and ankles. I recommend trying all formations to determine which one feels most supportive to you. Make sure your ankles do not hang off the props and both your knees and ankles are level with one another.

Either curl your arms in or stretch them out, placing one hand on top of the other.

This is the basic shape and what you can do if you only have a few props available.

More props? Let's build a cocoon.

Do all of the things noted above and add:

> A bolster or cushion at your back.
>
> A blanket under your bottom wrist.
>
> A block just outside of the place where your headrest is.
>> Set a bolster or cushion vertically on top of it. Bend your arm and rest it there.
>
> A blanket to cover your body.

Once You Are in It

Keep your eyes open. Notice the first 5 breaths just as they are. Then close your eyes. Scan your body from the top of your head to the tips of your toes, from the tips of your toes to the top of your head. Do this 3–5 times, allowing yourself to simply notice what you feel and where you feel it. Become aware that you are in a cocoon-like place and even allow yourself to consider that the "you" who set up this shape is not the one that is lying down. A transformation is already underway.

For the next several moments, pay attention to your breath. Gradually, invite your breath to become longer and steadier, nothing forced though. After the inhale, notice the pause. Breathe out as soon as you need to. We aren't holding the breath, only watching. Continue to breathe this way, paying attention to the inhale and the pause right after it for 5–7 breaths. Then shift your attention to noticing the exhale and the pause right after the exhale. Again, not holding the breath, forcing, or even creating a pause, but noticing the one that already exists. Repeat this for 5–7 cycles. Then shift to the exhale. Then notice the pause after. Exhale again. And notice the pause after again. Anchor your awareness in the pause more than the movement of the breath. Remember, you aren't holding the breath or forcing a pause. Do this as long as you want, until you feel your mind and body release.

You can also steady your awareness by quietly saying on the inhale "amazing" and on the exhale "grace."

Stay in the pose for 10–15 minutes.

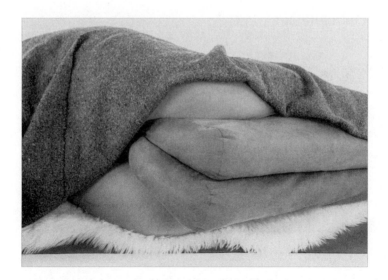

After the Pose

My favorite way to come out of this pose is slowing and starting by removing one prop, then pausing, then moving another, and then pausing, allowing myself to notice the shifts that occur as I remove the tangible support. Once all of the props are gone, I rest on my side in an unsupported fetal position for 10 or so breaths and ask myself, *What wisdom is present for me now?* It's usually a single word or phrase.

Come up to sitting and journal or draw for 2–3 minutes. Reconnect to the words "amazing grace." Hold *Pause, Rest, Be* at your heart. Open to a page. Allow the message you need to meet you now.

Considerations

1. If you are pregnant, practice this pose on your left side.
2. If you can't easily get up and down off the floor, try practicing this pose on your bed.
3. If you have a hard time settling in or being still, dance or move your body for 5–10 minutes before you rest.

The liminal is a spacious place and defined by its lack of definition. Insights and answers that come from the space between often surrender us to more questions. Questions that deserve answers. Questions that feel urgent though the answering of them cannot be rushed or forced.

In this section, I intentionally leave more open space and offer fewer words.

I invite you to start with Side-Lying pose and then return to the book.

Each time you return to this section, touch each page slowly. Silently read each word and then aloud. Be with this section one page at a time.

Yes, there are fewer words here. No less meaning, wisdom, or depth.

The answers and insights that come in liminal space have the power to change us in big and small ways. I have found that when I do not rush through such a place, what emerges shifts my course, every single time.

Being here, now, our course is taking on a different dimension and shape already.

Rest and allow.

You are not lost. You are here to reorient your way to the path that is truly yours to walk.

How many titles have you claimed? How many distinctions have you been given? How much of it felt unreal and false? Like you were wearing a suit that impressed everybody but it barely fit you? You are allowed to change as many times as you need to become your authentic self.

Forget your name and what they call you. You came here to remember your heart and soul.

There is no way to apply existing logic
here. There is no sense or meaning to make.
There is no normal to idealize and place on
a pedestal. There is only the ground you
are sitting on and even that feels like it is
crumbling. Sink into the ground. You are a
seed.

You can't muscle through this. This requires surrender. Surrender does not mean giving up. It is giving over. A giving over to something or someone with everlasting arms that you can lean into and be held by. Call in grace.

You are in an unfamiliar place. You meticulously packed your bags for the journey. You thought you had a map, compass, or guide. It turns out that you only have your senses. If that is all you have, trust. It is enough.

You are not alone. There are forces seen and unseen walking with you.

How to make friends with your fear:

Face it.

Look it in the eye.

Breathe with it.

Say, "Hello. How are you?

Why are you here right now?"

Listen to the answers.

Listen for what isn't being spoken. You know how fear likes to talk a lot of outrageous smack? What if you got curious about what fear isn't saying? What is fear leaving out of the story that you know is true?

The truth is that only the most courageous are ever brought this far and deep into the unknown. The ones who are willing to face the darkness within themselves and the world to understand the level of light needed to move forward. You are here because you are one of the courageous ones.

This is preparing you for what you asked for. Walking the road to your dream prepares you to arrive at it. To live it. To love it. To know how to greet it. To thrive within it.

Right now, the only light coming through is that of an intense fire—the fire of your rage. You do not have to simmer down. Do not burn yourself either. Peer into the fire. What fuels it? And how can the light of it serve you in this dark place?

When you examine your darkness, you see how much light is hidden behind it. You can't walk around it, only through. Going through creates friction. That friction rubs you until there is a whisper of shine. Avoiding your darkness dulls your light and silences the hum of your glow.

As you journey through, hum. Hum yourself a lullaby. Hum a prayer. Hum sounds of hope, love, despair, longing, and thanksgiving. Hum softly or loudly. Hum to remind yourself of the still, small light within.

Even if the world as you knew it was not the world you wanted it to be, you are allowed to mourn the death of it. You may have yearned for this divorce from that reality and still weep now as you stand at the grave of your marriage. Perhaps the life you were living wasn't the life you are worthy of and desired. You are allowed to grieve it as it disappears and becomes invisible. This is a threshold.

If you don't walk through the valley, you do not cultivate the capacity to make it to the peak. As you learn to be with your grief, you expand your capacity to be in your joy. If you cannot face your grief, you limit your access to joy. Grief and joy are sacred twins.

You do not have to face it all at once. Your heart is a portal—a doorway into the truth hidden underneath every feeling and emotion. Perhaps today, you sit outside the door and lean your back against it. And then, the next day, you crack open the door. And so on. You do not have to fling it open. Do not bolt it closed. Do not lock yourself out of your own heart.

Your heart may be broken. Walk through the opening. Rest in the inner sanctuary of your being. Place your most intimate, soft, and longing prayers on the altar within your heart. This is one way to remember you are whole.

You are being stripped down to your wholeness. The layers and baggage that you are shedding may feel like you are falling apart—shattering into pieces. Those pieces weren't yours. The things falling away never belonged to you. Let it all fall.

You are learning what is you and what is
not you, what is simply a habit, condition, or
thing you picked up along the way and forgot
to put down. You've worn some things so
long that you think it's really your skin. You
are learning what is yours and what is not
yours. You are shedding.

You may think you are not doing very much
at all. All of this shifting from the inside out.
All of this adjusting and readjusting to what
is. All of this releasing and letting go requires
energy. Transformation requires rest.

This is uncomfortable. You want to rush through. You want to hurry to whatever is next. Next is not available yet. Next is being made possible now, and it does not exist yet. Slow down and dream a little. You have the power to conjure and imagine what is next. This is a place of possibility.

Hold on to your faith and courage. Let everything else go. A change is coming.

Listen. It's time. Now. Spread your wings and take off to the sky. After all of this, nothing can harm you now. You know your song. Rise up singing. Rise.

A Prayer for Liminal Space

Goddess of the space in between,

We thank you for being the wild and beautiful ocean that you are. One that dwells between the shore of what was and what will be. One that connects us all to the place of our Ancestors and the source of our future. We thank you that your waves are unceasing in their devotion to moving us toward liberation. We enter into your blue-bellied womb before every beginning and after every ending. Let us not become trapped or caught up in the mystery and fear surrounding us. You who are not black or white. Day or night. Good or bad. When you come and swallow us in your luminous darkness, may we have the good sense to simply lie down, float for a while, and dream. Let us dream of something new and ancient. Let us dream of nothing and every-thing in altering time. Let us dream of composting old things and planting seeds that will grow for generations to come. Let us dream of boundlessness even when we feel stuck and small. Let us dream of another world. And after all of that, baptize us in possibility and allow the breath of your water to call us awake. With eyes wide open, we reach shore. We begin.

PART THREE

Beginnings

When now is a beginning—a tender and wide-eyed place.

It is a place where something or someone has arrived. Something worked for, prayed for, waited on. It is also a place of pain. A place with a past and history behind it. It is an unknown challenge to be faced. There is no beginning without an end, so it is a place where something has been lost, shifted, radically transformed, or fallen away.

Beginnings are humbling places. Sometimes we see and feel a beginning coming because many waves of endings have beat against the shore of our being. We have been worn down to scraps of sediment again and again. We understand there is nothing to do but start over. And sometimes we arrive in a new place, a beginning, after fumbling through the dark, disoriented, and adrift. We find ourselves at the beginning of a journey holding only ourselves. We look around, and everything is new. And then there are the joyous beginnings of new life, weddings, and dreams coming into reality.

We are in a communal birthing room. A baby is emerging, and there is no way to push her back in. Here we are, holding a naked, slippery, and crying *something* in our arms. Here we are, perhaps unexpectedly meeting ourselves in rare form after travailing, laboring, fighting, and surrendering, at times alone and in silence. At other times, with a community and through so much sweat and prayer. No matter the way, we've come to this point.

The communal birthing room is overflowing. There are wails of weariness. The kind that signifies unquenched thirst from mouths after long and treacherous travel. There are sounds of elation, clapping, and women shouting, as I have heard the mothers of the church say so many times, "Thank Yuh." *Thank Yuh* for making a way for me through a journey I didn't necessarily set out to take. *Thank Yuh* for the strength to surrender and let go. To let things end in order to begin again. *Thank Yuh* for bringing me from a mighty long way so that I can see a new day. *Thank Yuh* for second, third, and fourth chances. *Thank Yuh* for not forgetting me even when I forgot myself. *Thank Yuh* that all of those endings did not end me. I am still here. Thank yuh Lord, God, Ancestors, and Benevolent spirits who walk with us. Thank Yuh!

All beginnings start with a single step, wobble, or crawl. You may be half doubled over and holding the rail. Yet you made it. We made it.

Beloveds, there are so many beginnings being conceived, birthed, and hoping to rise through us. Do you feel it? Can you sense it? You've lost so much. You've put so much down. You can carry this. It is a seed. Can you nourish the seeds of this beginning within your own body, heart, and mind? I promise you I will do the same. And we will gather our seeds of hope, and we will plant them. We will take care of them. They will grow beyond possibility into reality. Will you kneel and bow with me? Will you offer up prayers to all that is righteous in the universe? Ask them to bless us all. Bless our seeds. May we grow and thrive. May we always have hope to begin again.

Let us end this journey called *Pause, Rest, Be* with beginning.

Child's Pose | Balasana

A Pose for Beginnings

The first power yoga class I ever took began with a Child's Pose. We took our knees just wide enough to fit our torso in between them, touched our big toes together, pushed our hips back, and brought our foreheads down to the ground. We stretched out our arms. As I pressed my forehead into the ground during that first Child's Pose, I was transported back to being a little girl.

Dressed in shaggy pajamas with my night bonnet to protect my braids on my head, I would kneel by my bedside along with my mama and sister. We would pray every night before going to bed. As a small girl, I did not know what to say. Mama would always say, "Ann," (that is what my family calls me) "you can say 'thank you' or tell God what is in your heart. Offer God your heart. He understands."

I would rarely say my prayers aloud. Yet as a child who was often bullied, called names, and grew up in poverty, what I would offer of my heart to God was this: *Thank you for helping me through this day. Please let tomorrow be a better day. A new begin-ning.* That first Child's Pose felt like a bedtime prayer with my mother and sister. A place to acknowledge what I was willing and longing to leave behind and offer my heart to The Divine as I started something new.

All of the years that I practiced power yoga, praying in a Child's Pose at the start of class became a personal ritual. Sometimes the prayer contained a lot of words. Many times, I would simply sigh and say, *Thank you for this place to begin again.*

———

Fast-forward a bit, and I attended my first restorative yoga class. I don't think I'd read the description. I just saw a class on the schedule and went. Keep in mind, at the time, I practiced power yoga at least five times a week. There were three other people present at this restorative yoga class, and everyone had at least six to eight different props. I turned up my nose at all of that "extra prop-having," threw my mat down, and sat on my one singular blanket.

The teacher was patient, kind, and generous. She brought me my other seven props and quietly said, "This class is about resting and being supported." I shrugged and thought, *I don't need all of that. I am strong.*

This restorative class began with a Child's Pose, except this time, we spent no less than five minutes setting up all of the props and held the actual pose for ten minutes. I spent the first few minutes deeply annoyed and thinking what a waste of time lying on a bunch of pillows and blankets and doing nothing was. I made to-do lists. I thought of all of the tasks I was not completing while I was in that class, supposedly resting. I wiggled. I fidgeted. I tossed. I turned. I gritted my teeth and tightened my jaw. I maybe even grumbled aloud at how slow, pointless, and annoying this "doing nothing" was.

Then something happened. My shoulders relaxed into the support beneath me. My jaw softened. My hips sank. My hands became heavy. My breath became a lullaby of whispers. Once again, I felt myself kneeling at a sacred altar and praying. This time, there were no words, only the feeling of being present, supported, carried even. My to-do list undid itself. I sighed and began to cry.

I cried because I realized how much I was carrying, doing, holding up, and holding on to. I cried because I realized I was really, really tired. That first Child's Pose in a power practice was the precursor to sweat, movement, posing, and working out. In this first restorative Child's Pose, I cried because I realized there was no place for me to go but in. I realized that "doing nothing" was about to bring me face-to-face with some real "ish" within. Softening required such inner strength. That first restorative class was destiny. It was the place where I realized the most transformative workout is within. It was a new beginning.

———

Salamba translates to "supported." *Bala* is a Sanskrit word that has several meanings: "young," "powerful," "strength of mind," and "childlike," among others. So *salamba balasana* means "supported child's pose." In Hinduism, the term appears most often when referring to youth, as in *bala Krishna* (young Krishna) and *Balasana* (Child's Pose). In more active styles of yoga, Balasana (Child's Pose) is a pose of respite from the movement, engagement, and doing. Even during more "physical" yoga, the layered meaning of *bala* comes into play. Indeed, there is a true strength of mind required to kneel in Child's Pose, to surrender to the need for a break, or to rest while everyone else is working. Child's Pose is a shape that transports us all the way back to our beginning.

———

I'd dreamed of owning my own yoga studio for so long, and the year my son was born proved to be the year that I finally had the courage to do it. But what happens when you arrive at your dream, you begin, and it's not the place you imagined? When the sweat, the blood, the sleep loss, the incantations, the offerings, the tears, and the sacrifice—none of it adds up? When all of that work doesn't yield enough to sustain you?

What happens when you can't remember why you started in the first place? What happens when your eyes are hazy, so you miss the clues sent to remind you? That first year of being a yoga studio owner, I questioned the stuff my dreams were made of. I unraveled and examined, thread by thread, the fabric upon which my vision was held.

The poet Langston Hughes once described living life with dying dreams as a bird whose wings have been broken.

Arriving at my dream cracked my wings and taught me the power in falling down, in kneeling.

The journey of arriving at the dream inevitably changes the dreamer. For me, that beginning, starting a business, brought me to my knees. So many days when I didn't know how I would make it to the next day as a start-up business owner and new mother, I'd find myself in a heap, swaddled in blankets, praying, crying, and resting in Child's Pose. So much has been born in the sacred space of Salamba Balasana: acceptance, letting go, resolve, discernment, faith, hope, trust, and the strength of mind to continue.

Ultimately, I have come to understand Child's Pose as the practice of remembering the womb and being born. Every beginning, big or small, is some kind of birth. In Child's Pose, we birth more acceptance of where we are and our growing process. Seeds of faith in the universal support that guides us begin to root and sprout within us. In Child's Pose, we recognize that for all we do not know, there is a cosmic knowing of our purpose beyond words, space, and time. The next one thousand steps may not be clear. But the next baby step comes into view as we bow in this sacred pose and place.

I've also learned that when we are particularly activated with the need to control, change, and fixate on every single little detail related to beginnings, it's best that we wrap ourselves in Balasana instead of simply setting up our bodies in the shape as we do in more active styles of yoga. Use props and allow support. In that way, we create a container to nourish, steady, and provide for us as we contract and expand into this beginning. Salamba Balasana.

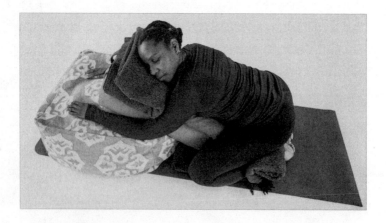

What You Need to Practice

A yoga mat, four blankets, two blocks, one bolster or couch cushion, two pillows, cozy socks, *Pause, Rest, Be,* a journal, and something to write with.

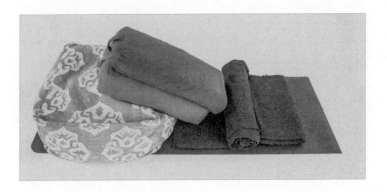

How to Set Up

TIME: 5–10 minutes

Create a landing place. Put down a yoga mat and layer on two blankets folded in half on top of your mat. This gives you a soft place to land. Take one block to its tallest level and one block four to six inches away from that block on the medium level.

Place your biggest bolster on top of the blocks. This should be at an angle. If the angle is too high, awkward, or uncomfortable, lower the blocks to the medium and lowest levels, respectively. Set one pillow at a 35- to 45-degree angle to the left and another to the right.

Place a blanket folded four ways at the top of the biggest bolster. It can support your head and neck if you need it to. Once you have all of these pieces set up, come to all fours in tabletop or kneeling position. Take your knees wide enough to nestle against the outside of the bolster. Bring your big toes together. Slowly move your hips back toward your heels.

They do not have to touch. In the process of moving your hips back, if you notice tightness or discomfort in your knees, roll up a blanket and place it in the crease behind your knees. Allow your torso to lie on the bolster. Rest your arms on the pillows to the left and right. If you feel chilly or would like a more wrapped and held feeling, ease out of the pose, drape the remaining blankets over your back (like a superhero cape), and return to the pose. Place your right ear down first and turn your head to the left at the halfway point of the hold.

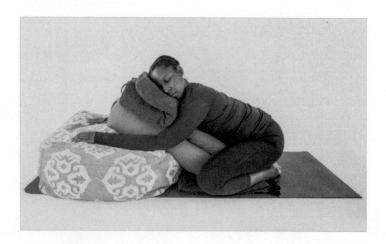

Once You Are in It

Slowly close your eyes. Scan your body from the top of your head to the tips of your toes, from the tips of your toes to the top of your head. Do this 3–5 times, allowing yourself to simply notice what you feel and where you feel it. Become aware that you are in a womb-like place, sustained, held, nourished, and completely supported. With each exhalation, allow the boundaries of this shape to even more fully hold each part of your body. With each exhalation, you let go of a layer of grasping, tension, constriction, worry, fear, dread, or whatever feels weighted, heavy, or immovable to you. Release.

Once you feel more connected to this place of sustenance, begin to notice your inhalation. We are simply noticing the breath, not controlling, shifting, or changing it—only noticing. Focus on your inhalation for 10–15 breaths. Then take your awareness to the center of your chest, your spiritual heart center. Follow your inhale as deep and far into your heart as possible. Sense that there is a back gate to your heart, and you may open it if you are ready. Your exhale carries you further into your heart. Remember, you are held in a sweet embrace, a kind of cosmic womb. Inhale, deep into your heart. Exhale even deeper into your heart, 10–15 breaths. Then allow your awareness to rest within your heart. A prayer or intention for your beginnings easily emerges from the deepest place within your heart as you rest. Offer up that prayer/intention.

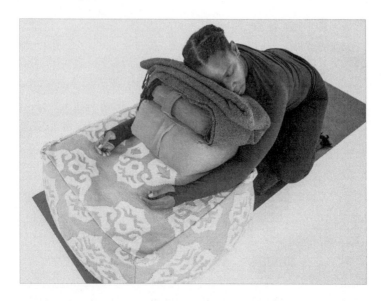

Stay in the pose for 5–10 minutes. When coming out, bring your chin to the center and curl your toes. Very gently press into your hands and lift your torso. Slowly stretch each leg out one at a time. Come to sitting quietly in the center of your mat or against a wall. You may sit straight-legged or cross-legged. Do what feels most comfortable.

After the Pose

As we slowly move out of Salamba Balasana, or Supported Child's Pose, we intentionally return and explore our body, heart, and mind with curiosity and awareness that something has been released and something else has arrived. This is the place to begin.

Journal or draw for 2–3 minutes. Reconnect to your intention or prayer. Hold *Pause, Rest, Be* at your heart. Open to a page. Allow the message you need for support moving forward to find you.

Considerations

If you have a hard time settling in or being still, do one of the following before you rest:

1. Turn on your favorite song with drums and bass tones in it and dance. You may start moving at any pace, then gradually slow down until you come to an organic stop.
2. Shake. Like, yes. Literally, shake your body. Start by shaking your feet, then swirling your hips. Next, shake your hands. Shake your whole body. Same as above, you may start shaking at any speed, then gradually slow down until you come to an organic stop.
3. Feel into the place in your body that is least settled or able to be still. Ask that place how it needs to move. Move the way it needs you to for 5–10 minutes.

12

Eyes on the Promise

The first person in my family to attend and finish college was my big cousin Tracy D. Norman. He went to a historically Black college, Savannah State University. I remember him leaving home with a trunk and backpack. He would come back for the holidays with Bob Marley and Sade tapes. I wanted to go where he was going, even though I didn't quite know how to get there.

Eventually, I figured it out, and I went to college. I walked in my cousin's footsteps, just in a slightly different direction. I went "up north" to Northeastern University in Boston. Much like him, I left home with very little in possessions, money, or even awareness of what it would take to live and be that far away from everything I had known.

I remember the ride from my hometown of Gainesville, Georgia, to Boston, Massachusetts. I sat looking out the window as the lush green and thick trees of my childhood slowly transformed into little hungry-looking things that seemed like I could wrap my whole hand around them. I witnessed rolling hills of red clay become gray, concrete skylines. As we crossed the line that separates the North from the South, the Mason-Dixon, and as the world outside my window changed, I changed.

My eighteen-year-old sense of "I'm ready for anything!" shifted to the feeling of one million fireflies fighting to keep their little light ablaze in my belly. My eyes became weeping muscadines of bittersweet streams pouring from me. *Where was I headed? What exactly was I doing? Would I be okay? Would I make it? What caused me to come this far away for school?* This beginning was wrapped up in pride, promises, and also pain.

Even as I was traveling to a place where thousands of others were beginning college, I felt alone. Mama sat in the front seat of the van, having her own experience of this beginning. No doubt feeling the weight of her prayers that brought this moment into being. Maybe even questioning herself and those prayers.

We journeyed on. There was nowhere else to go but forward despite the buzzing in my belly and the tears in my eyes. Through the storm of my emotions, I recalled the end of college for my cousin Tracy. I remembered his graduation. I remembered the sense of collective achievement and joy that one of us had "made it." I remembered the celebration and certainty that came from seeing him walk across the stage. If he could do it, so could I. Looking back for just a moment gave me the courage to face the beginning with my eyes on the promise even as I felt my way through the pain of leaving so much behind. And so I journeyed on. There was nowhere else to go but forward.

May you journey on. There is no place to go but forward.

Take a moment to look back and reflect on a beginning that held both promise and pain for you. In looking back, what do you see, feel, and understand now that you didn't then? How can you carry that wisdom forward toward whatever beginning you may be facing now?

13

Stumbling Is the Way

We don't just start out walking or even crawling. We start as round lumps of earthen clay that must be held, carried, tended to, and allowed to take shape and form. If my memory serves me correctly, my son's pathway to walking was this:

Kicking, wiggling, rolling over, sliding, scooting, one-knee crawling, two-knee crawling, pulling up, lots of falling—so much falling. Finally, he took his first wobbly, uncertain, yet sure steps. Uncertain because it was new, unfamiliar, a modality he had no experience in. Sure, because by any means, he was going to get to the little squishy blue ball that my friend Tabby held out in front of him. He didn't quite know the *how*. He had to stumble, trip, roll around, cry out in frustration, resist support, get back up, fall again, and cry for support again and again.

Yet, the *what* was apparent, known, and visible. Move toward the person smiling while both inching backward and reaching their hands forward. Knowing the *what* was enough. It didn't matter how many times his sense of balance seemed to betray him; he trusted his feet. He trusted his ten little toes. He had faith in the *what* to reveal the way, the how. And when he was tired, he'd sit down, play, rock, or drink milk.

There my friend was: inching backward with the shiny object as my son reached, moved, and wobbled forward—one shaky step. Two steps and his legs buckled a little, and then he pushed them straighter. Three . . . four . . . five . . . ten steps, and he'd gone beyond what I thought was his goal and motivation—to get to the shiny ball. I think he and I both realized this movement beyond the "goal" at the same time because he stopped. He looked at me. Then he stood up tall, lifted his hands, and clapped.

He didn't fret over when or how he would walk. He moved with curiosity about the possibilities that existed in his feet. He only learned because he had plenty of space to stumble and fall.

In my very adult-ish life, I've learned to judge many things by the way they start. When I start things and it's not smooth, perhaps there are a few fits and stutters, I'll think, *Oh, this is a bad sign.* I'll begin my projections and sometimes even conclude, *Might as well quit now, if this is the way it's beginning.* Or worse still, I will deny myself new beginnings and starts because I am not already "good" at it.

Stumbling is the way we learn to walk. Persist.

What is something you've always wanted to do or try, but you haven't because you think you'll look silly, people will laugh, or you fear you won't be "perfect" at it? Can you commit to trying it within the next three days or sooner?

14

Noways Tired

It was Saturday, March 13, 2020. For me, that was the day the reality hit me in the gut, face, and heart that we were in a pandemic. It was that day I realized we were at the beginning of something we had never seen. I was leading a yoga teacher training. It was the last weekend of the training, and ultimately, the last moment I taught a group of people in my yoga studio, Sacred Chill West. On that day, while we sat in a circle, facing a canyon of unknown proportions, a student asked me how I felt about all that was going on.

I inhaled, and the word I exhaled and spoke was "brave."

Brave, not because I had things stored, coffers, a stash, or anyone/institution/system to come to my rescue as we faced a pandemic.

Brave, not as if there wasn't a single fear rattling me awake each night because there was.

Brave, not because, somehow, I knew my business, Sacred Chill West, would still be standing after it all. It actually didn't.

Brave because of what I had already lived through:

> Hunger
> Food, clothes, and housing insecurity
> Lack of access to an equitable and safe education
> Limited means of transportation
> Rationing of everyday "essentials:" soap, toilet paper,
>   toothpaste, hot water
> Unreliable consistency in utilities

I could go on. This was part of my childhood reality despite my mother working two jobs and me working as early as fourteen years old.

I come from a forgotten place. At the beginning of the global shutdown in the United States in 2020, I remembered this and my capacity to face reality head-on opened up.

Sometimes beginnings are beautiful, exciting, and wanted. Other times, we encounter a beginning that looks and feels like total destruction. In those moments, remember. Remember what you have risen from and walked through. There's a gospel song by James Cleveland and Curtis Burrell that I love. The title is "No Wayz Tired." The words, "I don't feel no ways tired. / I've come too far from where I started from. / Nobody told me the road would be easy. / I don't believe he brought me this far to leave me."

This song calls me to honor that all of my experiences have prepared me to stand where I am no matter how light or dark. It restores my faith in rest as Divine fuel that, when taken, supports me in feeling "noways tired."

When you are at the beginning of a road that doesn't look easy, pause and reflect.

You've walked hard roads before. You've gotten lost before. You've hobbled on before. You've made it through before.

I don't believe he | she | it brought us this far to leave us.

Know this and be brave.

Take three minutes to make a list of all the ways that you've been brave before. Take a few more moments to write a list of times you've made it through, no matter how challenging. When you face a new beginning that appears to be a hard road ahead, remember.

15

The Underbelly

We can tuck and hide so much to make ourselves "more lovable" until we confine the parts of us that need the most light, the most real love, the most nourishment—to a dark corner of our being.

One day while breathing, meditating, and repeating "I can. I will. I must deeply love and nourish myself," a little voice of wisdom said, "Self-love is this."

My hand was literally at my underbelly, the place that has morphed into discolored, loose, and scarred skin since giving birth. The place that already had so many war markings before that.

"This?" I silently ask. "Not this—no one loves this."

Voice of wisdom. "Yes, this. Absolutely this. This is your way to self-love."

Self-love is seeing fully, with tenderness and compassion, that part of ourselves that we have learned to believe is most unworthy of being seen, unlovable, or flawed.

It is accepting, touching, feeling, tending to, singing to, gazing completely at the place that others have turned their eyes away from.

It is wanting what has been unwanted within us.

It is holding our underbelly, or wherever that place is that we've experienced "no one loves this."

It is holding and loving that part of ourselves. That is just the beginning.

What place within you are you just beginning to love? What place within you do you believe is still untouchable, unlovable, or in need of hiding? How can you reveal more of that place to yourself?

16

A Warrior's Welcome

A while back, I read something regarding postpartum women in another culture from a bygone time.

The article noted that, for weeks after giving birth, the mother was mothered and her primary role was to connect to and nurture her baby. The women of the village tended to her so that she and the baby could begin and thrive (not simply survive) through the fourth trimester, or time immediately following giving birth.

Once that time ended, the new mother and her baby would go back to the village. When they reentered society, they were given a warrior's welcome.

This struck me: a warrior's welcome.

A warrior's welcome acknowledges that even in the most peaceful birthing processes, there is a kind of inner fight present.

To bring forth something new, we all must slay our inner and outer beasts, dip into our own valley, climb rugged mountains, and face Goliath with the triple slingshot of skill, strength, and surrender.

In birthing a child, one's body expands and is broken open so that the circle of humanity and our lineage is not broken. In labor, one pours her heart over a clothed pew lined with trillions of raw threads: spools of hope, anticipation, expansion, contraction, longing, fear, doubt, and triumph.

A warrior's welcome acknowledges that after the creation and creative process, we are not the same. We have a new knowing, essence, and capacity. We have burned and risen. We have fallen apart and come together.

Honor the times and places you have given birth. Times you have peeled back your old self, reached through generations of beliefs, muscle, stories, and blood to retrieve a deeper truth from the memory of your soul in order to live with more purpose.

Who but a warrior can do all of that and live to tell about it?

⁓

We all give birth to a multitude of things and in a plethora of ways, children or not. What have you gestated, labored for, and delivered into your life that was a battle requiring skill, strength, and discernment to know when to let go? Sit quietly. Recall these times, and at each memory, silently say to that version of yourself, "Welcome home, Warrior."

17

Breaking Code

In the middle of an argument, he looked at me, enraged, and said, "You don't want a man. You want a dog. You want someone to jump and run at your command. You are asking too much. You are saying too much. What real man is gonna deal with you and all of your questions, huh? Not me!"

I was young and "in love." This was his response to me bringing up my discomfort with his perpetual lateness for our dates and his unwillingness to be transparent about where he was. I had no answer. I went radio silent as he gunned the engine of his car and recklessly sped up. We were clearly going nowhere. At twenty, I desperately wanted this person to love me for me. Me: an intelligent, nonconforming, generous, kind woman who fiercely loved, respected, elevated, and rooted for women in a world that systemically just didn't do that. A womanist.* Yet, I also hid the woman I was in order to fit into his worldview. A view that was not just informed by family or even culture but society.

That argument didn't begin in that car. I grew up watching powerful and brilliant women be devalued, "put in their place," and undermined in the worst ways in families, workplaces, communities, and places of worship. It's an argument that stretches back across space and time. One that happens with and without words across the world. One that sadly too often happens with fists, threats, and in a ruthless cycle. One that happens in boardrooms, backrooms, and bedrooms. The center of the argument was held together by two shaky pillars. One pillar, "A real man doesn't have to be accountable to anyone or anything, especially a woman." Another pillar, "A good woman better keep quiet, not ask too many questions, and just ride

---

* Definition by Alice Walker, *In Search of Our Mothers' Gardens: Womanist Prose* (New York: Houghton Mifflin Harcourt, 1983), xi: "*Womanist*: From *womanish*. (Opp. of 'girlish,' i.e., frivolous, irresponsible, not serious.) A black feminist or feminist of color. From the black folk expression of mothers to female children, 'you acting womanish,' i.e., like a woman. Usually referring to outrageous, audacious, courageous, or willful behavior. Wanting to know more and in greater depth than is considered 'good' for one. Interested in grown-up doings. Acting grown up. Being grown up. Interchangeable with another black folk expression: 'You trying to be grown.' Responsible. In charge. Serious. . . . Loves music. Loves dance. Loves the moon. *Loves* the Spirit. Loves love and food and roundness. Loves struggle. *Loves* the Folk. Loves herself. *Regardless*."

along." In silence, I sat between these columns that threatened to hold me in place. I wondered, *Do I value myself? Do I let this person tell me who I am supposed to be? Do I choose him over me? Do I choose him over me?*

We sped along, going nowhere. We reached a stop sign, and that was the signal and message I needed that day. I got out of the car and began to walk. It was cold and almost dark. The only light guiding me was the blaze of my conviction. A fire, really. A fire that was fueled by a lifetime of beliefs, stories, and even sermons about what a woman could or shouldn't ask for and do. Even as the sun was setting, the radiance of truth was dawning in me. *I didn't come to this planet to live in any man's shadow, simply ride "shotgun," or allow anyone to dictate my "place."*

When we step beyond the tremulous pillars of deeply rooted belief systems, when we get out of the car, when we walk away from something so old that we've been mindlessly believing it's *just that way,* only then can we chart a new course. A new way is created one uncomfortable step at a time, one challenging choice that refuses to honor the status quo at a time.

Institutional oppression is encoded in our most intimate relationships, including the one we have with Self. I broke a code that night when I left the shelter of the car and walked away into the wild of the evening. I laid a rotting belief to rest and moved right over it. He and those already-shaky posts holding a debilitated and old system up began to crack. The cracking began within me and rippled out as I slammed the door.

I refuse to spend my life and relationships holding up beliefs that create harm for me and others. Every step I take, I write a new code. May all women be free.

What code, belief, or way of being were you intimately raised with that you are beginning to realize creates pain for you and others? What is one action you can take that interrupts it or begins to chip away at its power in your personal life?

18

Questions and Answers

My first job out of college was teaching middle-school reading, writing, and math. I moved across the country from Boston to Phoenix to teach via Teach for America. Somehow, I put everything I owned into two or three suitcases and simply went. Some part of my brain shielded me from spiraling into the place of fretting and thinking this was a big deal until I was almost there. I looked out over the rich, orange, and sunset haze of everything in the desert, and a feeling of complete terror descended on me as the plane began to land. The gravity of my new role, *teacher*, glued me to my seat as we touched down, and everyone else immediately unclicked their seat belt, stood up, and got ready to go. I was not ready. I thought over and over and over, *I am not ready for this new job, this new place, this new responsibility.* I clung to the safety of my chair for as long as I could. I was the last one off the plane, and I walked slowly, picked up my luggage, and headed out into the ripe, hot Southwest air.

I had been so excited when I applied for the job. I was confident and present during the interview. When I received my acceptance package, I was overjoyed. And now that the moment had actually arrived, I was ready to quit before I even started. So many questions arose. *Can I do this job? Why did I think this was a good idea, again? What if I fail? What if my students fail? What have I gotten into?* I almost dismissed the questions and then decided to sit with each one as if it were an old and trusted friend versus a stranger to be ignored and rejected.

Each question pointed toward my care about the work I was embarking on. Each question required and was worthy of an honest answer. An honest answer that didn't arrive from the part of me that was fearful, scared, tired from traveling, and untrusting of this stage of the process because it was new. But the part of me that applied, interviewed, and saw every single step before this final one through. The questions were not there to taunt me, fill me with doubt, or even test me. They were there to remind me of my why. They were there to affirm for me that I was where I needed and wanted to be. As long as I continued to show up, I could live the answers, one day at a time.

Make a list of questions you have about your current job or work. Questions that, based on your perception or experiences, may have indicated only doubt and fear. Is there another way to see the questions? What is that way?

19

A Desire Started

Something made you roll your eyes, hiss a little, and think, *They are so extra—ugh*, as you scrolled through their feed or timeline.

Is there someone you feel like you are silently in competition with?

Is there someone you watch and might even take notes from, but you don't "follow," "like," or "heart" them?

We know that social media has created a means to constantly compare that never existed before. And we know that comparing ourselves to someone else's parts will always ensure we feel like we are coming up short and can never be enough.

Yet. Still.

Can we learn something from compassionately examining who and what we envy?

I'll share a personal experience that I've tucked away and carried around for a while.

Before I became a mama, I'd suck my teeth when people talked about, posted about, wrote about, or shared pictures of their kids. Or I'd pretend to be overly interested. Once, while on a retreat, a woman kept talking about her children. At first, I was *so* into it. But it seemed to go on too long. My faux interest turned to pure irritation. I said to her, "Girl . . . I thought you came here to rest and be free of them and all that. Don't you have something else in your life to talk about?" (Yes, y'all, I said that to someone). I was so annoyed at her.

Was it annoyance? Was it *at* her? I went, sat with my feelings, and examined my response. Annoyance gave way to the feeling of a sharp rock in my belly. My heart felt punctured open and like a 1,000-miles-per-hour wind howled through it.

I held myself and wrapped deep breaths around my spirit. Then it happened.

This feeling was a tunnel to crawl and peer through. A way to both see and humbly touch what I wanted—that I desired so deeply, but was afraid to admit it for fear that it wouldn't or couldn't happen.

I wanted children that I would miss on a retreat. I wanted to unroll my yoga mat and have little socks that had been left behind fall out. I wanted to have snacks and toys in my bag just in case the munchies descended upon my munchkin. I wanted to love someone without conditions the way it seemed like this mother did her children. I wanted to be loved that way.

For many reasons, I couldn't and wouldn't admit that longing any other way. And so that thing, that big desire, dressed up like annoyance and strolled in as envy. Only once fully investigated did it reveal something I'd meticulously hidden and covered up beneath other emotions, interests, busyness, and even ambitions.

Envy does not feel good and is not "nice." No one wants to admit to it. The truth is: it is often a determined guide and teacher.

Looking our envy in the eye can show us what we really want and haven't been brave and honest enough to name.

Who or what do you envy? What longing or desire might be asking you to take notice through this fiery emotion? And most importantly, what are you going to do about it?

20

Forever, One Day at a Time

A wedding is a beautiful ritual and rite of passage. For me, it wasn't the beginning of my marriage. My marriage began the day I woke up, gasped, and thought to myself, "This needs to end." It was the day after our two-year anniversary party, a time when the full honeymoon began to wane, wax, and crest. *This needs to end* occurred to me as I watched my husband do what he does every morning: stand in the closet, scratch his beard, check his paper calendar that hangs on the wall, and then grab his clothes before heading to the shower. *This needs to end* was the beginning of a realization I'd held at bay. The realization that *Wait. What? This is forever ever? Forever ever?*

I was having a grown moment. I didn't want to commit to forever anymore. I didn't want to know this morning routine like the back of my hand. I didn't want to share space with a beard-scratching person who was always here.

Or did I? I was two years into a marriage that was joyful, steady, growing, and nourishing when I started to freak out on the inside. Before this relationship, I'd conformed to "situationships" that were dysfunctional, unreliable, and so wrong that the right feeling in my marriage felt off to me. I knew how to deal with unsteady, inconsistent, and even disloyal. Two years into marriage was when an alarm began to sound saying *No* to this goodness. *No* to this knowing. *No* to this consistent presence. *Noooo.*

What do we do when our past demons have a choke hold on us and say *this needs to end* at the beginning of something so right, it feels wrong? We listen. We get curious. We ask questions. We investigate what's true. We go to therapy. We come out of hiding. We dismantle and put ourselves back together. We pay attention to what's beneath the surface. Sometimes new is so different, we crave a regression back to the old.

I am grateful for the part of me that knew this relationship, this one, this is a yes. We are more than a decade into forever and what I understand now is that forever is built one day at a time.

What or who is new in your life right now? How does it feel?

21

Forgive Yourself First

I recently began a new decade of life and wrote a letter to my twenty-year-old self. Here's what I said to her:

> If you do not love yourself, flaws and all, it doesn't matter who else says they love you. You will not believe them. You will pull them into your irreverence for yourself. They will see how you treat you. They will take notes.
>
> The best of them will simply walk away and remember how beautiful, smart, and fierce they thought you could be. The worst of them will break your heart and teach you new ways to do the same. You accept the love you believe that you deserve.
>
> Can I tell you, sweetheart, you deserve so much devotion, compassion, deep love? Someone who will not leave you even when the night is long and the valley is deep. That someone is you. You deserve yourself.

Your life is worth fighting for. Thank you for deciding that if you could just make it to one class, then the next, then the next, you could keep living.

In the words of Rayya Elias, "The truth has legs; it always stands. When everything else in the room has blown up or dissolved away, the only thing left standing will always be the truth. Since that's where you're gonna end up anyway, you might as well just start there."*

You don't have to play nice. You only have to be real.

Be courageous enough to hold your father's hands, look him in the eye, and say, "We can't begin again. We can't erase yesterday. We can start where we are right now. Are you willing to do that?" Be wise enough to be honest with him. You don't have as much time with him as you think.

It is not a mistake if you learn and carry the lesson with you. Even if you don't do that, forgive yourself first.

What would you say to yourself ten or twenty years ago? Write your previous self a letter and then read it to them out loud. Listen.

---

* Catie L'Heureux, "*Eat, Pray, Love* Author Elizabeth Gilbert's Partner Rayya Elias Has Died," *The Cut*, January 5, 2018. https://www.thecut.com/2018/01/eat-pray-love-author-elizabeth-gilbert-mourns-rayya-elias-death.html.

22

Keep on Stepping

His mouth moved in slow motion. Did the room shrink? Maybe it expanded? Was I being squeezed tight? Was I free falling?

I did my best to listen as he spoke.

My heart slowed down. Everything else sped up.

Weighted bombs hurled from his mouth.

Cancer. Aggressive. Treatment. Must. Start. Soon.

That's when Birdie Mae Moon entered the room of my mind and heart. She stood there steady and with all of the confidence in me and the universe. She held my hand and whispered to me, "Okay, I am here. Now, what's our next step? And the step after that? And the step after that? We know how to do this. One foot in front of the other and keep on stepping. One step in front of the other and keep on stepping."

When my beloved mother-in-law was diagnosed with cancer, went through months of grueling treatments, and finally came out on the other side of it all, she shared this truth with me. That her grandmother, Birdie Mae Moon, who passed decades ago and is an Ancestor now, walked with her through the process.

As she began the treatment process, her courage came from remembering how her grandmother always believed in her. She summoned wisdom and faith from her spirit and memory.

Her ability to continue resided in the awareness that she only needed to take one step at a time and devote herself to that.

In facing the beginning of a life-changing diagnosis, health challenge, or illness, we are called into the truth and power of a single step. Resolving to "keep on" from the start supports us. Yet, getting ahead of ourselves slows us down.

One step.

It might be sedated, trembling, and heavy.

One step.

That step might require that we lean on somebody else's arm. That arm might be someone we've always held up: a partner, a daughter, a son, a sister, a brother, or a coworker.

Just one step.

That arm may be the everlasting arm of a grandmother who has left this earth yet promised she would never leave us.

One step.

And so, we face what must be faced with eyes that belong to the stream of time. We see those who are behind us and within us. We see those who are inside of us and yet to come. We see that we are both confined to and free to take only a single step at a time.

One step.

There may be immense pain, disorientation, uncertainty, fear, worry, despair, dread, rage, blame, regret, longing, and resistance as we begin and continue.

One step.

We may feel like we know nothing.

One step, though.

Just one step.

We are never alone.

Love will come in full force and step with us.

Love will carry us when we can't carry ourselves.

The Grandmothers will hold our hearts and hands along the way.

The road to recovery and healing may be lined with both ravishing fire and ice.

Still, it's "One step. Then, one step. Okay. Now, rest, child. Rest. Don't you get weary. One step. Here we go. One step." It's Grandmother Birdie Mae Moon's sacred whisper, "Keep on stepping. Keep on stepping."

A Prayer for All of Our Beginnings

Great Spirit of beginnings,

Thank you for meeting us here. We ask you to bless our beginnings and fill the way ahead with grace, ease, and space to rest for a spell of time. We've come a mighty long way to start. We promise to remember who and what came before us. To honor the lessons from the roads we've traveled. Teach us to not despise our beginnings even if they are humble as dirt, because all good and worthy things rise up from the ground. Every blossom was once a tiny little thing in need of sunlight and water, just like us. We pour libations from the back of our eyes onto the altar of this beginning. We create a stream that stretches through the world and doesn't let us forget that every minute someone exhales for the last time as someone inhales for the first time.

From the pulpit of our hearts, we lift our voices toward The Divine sanctuary of your ear.

We dig down into our souls to offer up this old hymn as we face something brand new:

> *Take my hand*
> *Lead me on, let me stand*
> *Through the storm, through the night*
> *Lead me on to the light*
> *Take my hand*
> *Lead me home.*

No matter where you find yourself, I pray you have the courage to pause sometimes. To rest and look within. To be still and know that you are not lost. You are making your way home.

Welcome home.

About the Author

Octavia Raheem is a mother, author of *Gather*, activist, and an experienced yoga teacher and practitioner. She began practicing yoga in 1999 and has been teaching since 2007. She founded Starshine & Clay, an online and retreat space for Black, Indigenous, and Women of Color to rest and restore. Born and raised in Gainesville, Georgia, her spirituality encompasses the universe and is very much anchored in the heart and soul of the sacred community she was raised in: Greater Timber Ridge Baptist Church.

Octavia has a distinctive voice. One that is wise, otherworldly, and also familiar. Her teaching is grounded in her roots and real-life experience as a woman learning to love herself as well as center her well-being and transformation via yoga, rest, meditation, and Yoga Nidra.

Her words are a glowing fire that everyone can gather around.